CHAPTER ONE

Introduction to Ciprofloxacin

What is Ciprofloxacin?

Ciprofloxacin is a synthetic antibiotic, chemically related to quinolone, generally indicated for most bacterial infections. The fluorine atom at the C6 position gives better antibacterial activity. This drug is broad-spectrum, which means virtually all Gram-positive and Gram-negative bacteria are sensible to it.

This antibiotic was introduced in the 1980s and quickly became one of the most widely prescribed antibiotics in the world due to its relatively high efficiency, primarily against Gram-negative pathogens. It is used to treat a wide variety of infections: respiratory, urinary, gastrointestinal systems; skin, bones, and other diseases.

Mechanism of Action

Ciprofloxacin was the first oral fluoroquinolone to be approved for human use. Mechanism of action This agent binds to the bacterial enzyme DNA gyrase and topoisomerase IV, thereby interfering with bacterial DNA transformation and transcription. DNA gyrase causes rapid negative supercoiling of the DNA strand, which is an important step during the initiation of the DNA replication and transcription process. Topoisomerase IV is required during cell division for separation of daughter DNA strands.

Ciprofloxacin inhibits these enzymes that do not enable the bacteria to replicate their DNA; because of this, the growth of the bacteria is stopped, and the bacterial cells die. Such a mode of action makes ciprofloxacin a potent bactericidal agent against many significantly replicating bacteria.

Pharmacokinetics

Ciprofloxacin is administered in three ways: orally, intravenously, and ophthalmically. There are differences in the pharmacokinetics depending on the route of administration.

The disposition of ciprofloxacin from the gastrointestinal tract after oral administration is rapid; oral bioavailability is around 70-80%. Food will delay its absorption slightly but not greatly affect the overall bioavailability. Ciprofloxacin is widely distributed in the body after absorption. High concentrations are achieved in the urinary tract, lungs, liver, gallbladder, and tissues of the body. The penetration of the cerebrospinal fluid is also high, and therefore, the drug can be used in treating meningitis.

Ciprofloxacin is not metabolized well in the liver. Only 10% to 20% of the drug is metabolized to inactive substances. The major metabolites are desethylene-ciprofloxacin and sulfociprofloxacin.

Most of the drug is excreted unchanged in the urine. From the administered dose, about 40-50% is eliminated in the first 24 hours. A minute percentage is excreted in the feces.

Spectrum of Activity

The antibiotic ciprofloxacin works against a large number of bacterial species due to the wide spectrum of its activity. Some of the common bacteria that are susceptible to cipro include:

Gram-negative bacteria: Escherichia coli, Pseudomonas aeruginosa, Haemophilus influenzae, Klebsiella pneumoniae, Enterobacter species, Neisseria gonorrhoeae, and Salmonella species.

Gram-positive bacteria: Staphylococcus aureus (including methicillin-resistant strains), Streptococcus pneumoniae, and Bacillus anthracis.

Atypical pathogens: Chlamydia pneumoniae, Mycoplas.

Although this is a wide spectrum, ciprofloxacin is less active against anaerobic bacteria and some Gram-positive organisms, like Streptococcus pyogenes and Enterococcus faecalis. Resistance to the drug, therefore, has developed in some strains of these organisms, limiting the use of ciprofloxacin in some instances.

Clinical Applications of Ciprofloxacin

Ciprofloxacin is indicated in a number of respiratory tract infections, mainly caused by Gram-negative organisms. These include:

Ciprofloxacin is not labeled as first-line therapy for community-acquired pneumonia. However, it does have activity against some of the atypical pathogens, like Legionella pneumophila and Mycoplasma pneumoniae. It can be used in patients with a beta-lactam or macrolide allergy.

Ciprofloxacin is often part of a combined regimen with other antibiotics for the treatment of HAP, more so if caused by multidrug-resistant Gram-negative organisms like Pseudomonas aeruginosa. It can be administered to those patients whose COPD is suspected to be exacerbated due to bacterial infection, especially if the offending pathogen is Haemophilus influenzae or Pseudomonas aeruginosa.

The significant penetration of ciprofloxacin into the urinary tract and the activity against the common uropathogens make it a drug of choice in the treatment of UTI.

Ciprofloxacin is effective against Escherichia coli, the most frequently isolated pathogen in uncomplicated UTIs.

In complicated UTIs, ciprofloxacin holds its position for management, for example, in the situation of a urinary catheter, structural abnormalities, or infection with a resistant organism. Ciprofloxacin is also approved for use in its treatment due to its appropriately high concentrations in renal tissue.

Typhoid fever; caused by Salmonella typhi, ciprofloxacin stands as one of the antibiotics in typhoid fever therapy, particularly in cases of resistance to other antibiotics in extended areas.

Ciprofloxacin is effective in treating various bacterial pathogens involving infectious diarrhea, such as Shigella and Campylobacter species.

Ciprofloxacin is a possible treatment for skin and soft tissue infections, particularly those caused by Gram-negative bacteria. Some of the examples are:

Even though it is considered a secondary, alternate drug, ciprofloxacin can be used in cases of cellulitis related to Gram-negative bacteria or in subjects allergic to penicillin.

Alone or combined with other antibiotics, Ciprofloxacin is sometimes used in some diabetic foot infections, especially when the cause is thought to be by Gram-negative bacteria such as Pseudomonas aeruginosa.

Ciprofloxacin is used in the therapy of osteomyelitis, or bone infection, and in septic arthritis, or joint infection, especially if Gram-negative, as in the case of Pseudomonas aeruginosa. Its penetration into bone and its broad-spectrum activity make it useful in these severe infections.

Dosage and Administration

Ciprofloxacin is supplied in these various dosage forms for clinical application:

Tablets for oral use: 250 mg, 500 mg, and 750 mg

Extended release tablets: 500 mg and 1000 mg for once-a-day dosing

Intravenous (IV) solution: It is indicated in the case of severe infections in general it requires higher concentrations of the drug more quickly than required.

Ophthalmic solution: to remove eye infections

Otic solution: to remove ear infections

The dosage of ciprofloxacin depends on the type of infection: bone/joint, intra-abdominal, systemic infections, and infections other than the urinary tract.

The following dosages are considered typical for a particular infection:

Respiratory Tract Infections

For mild-to-moderate infection:
500 mg orally every 12 hours

For severe infection:
750 mg orally every 12 hours
or
400 mg IV every 8-12 hours
  Uncomplicated: 250-500 mg PO q12h.
  Complicated: 500 mg PO q12h or 400 mg IV q12h.

Pyelonephritis: 500 mg PO q12h or 400 mg IV q12h.

Gastrointestinal infections:

Traveler's diarrhea: 500 mg PO q12h for 3 days.

Typhoid fever: 500 mg PO q 12 h x 10-14 days.

Skin and soft tissue infections :

Mild to moderate: 500 mg PO q 12 h

Severe: 750 mg PO q12h or 400 mg IV q12h

Bone and joint infections :

500-750 mg PO q12h or 400 mg IV q12h x 4-6 wk

Special Populations

Renal impairment: The dose of ciprofloxacin should be adjusted in patients with reduced renal function to avoid its accumulation and likely toxicity. In patients with creatinine clearance of 30-50 mL/min, a 50% dose reduction was recommended. In those with a creatinine clearance of less than 30 mL/min, the dose is reduced by 75%.

Hepatic impairment: Dose adjustment is generally not required in mild and moderate degrees of hepatic impairment patients; patients with severe hepatic impairment require caution.

Pediatric patients: Ciprofloxacin is not considered appropriate except in the case of life-threatening medical conditions when no tolerable alternatives are available. For FDA-approved indications, the dosage is 10-15 mg/kg every 12 hours, and the maximum dose must not exceed 500mg per dose.

Geriatric patients: Elderly patients may experience an increased vulnerability to the adverse effects of ciprofloxacin, particularly tendon rupture. Dosage adjustments are required according to renal function.

Adverse Effects and Warnings

Ciprofloxacin is, for most part, well-tolerated. As with any other medicine, it may sometimes lead to certain side effects. Some common side effects include:

Gastrointestinal disturbances: The usual side effects are nausea, diarrhea, vomiting, and abdominal pain. These are generally mild and brief but may be disturbing in a few patients.

Central nervous system effects: The incidence of headache, dizziness, and insomnia is relatively high. More serious CNS effects, including seizures, hallucinations, and tremors, are rare but do occur, especially in those with underlying CNS disorders.

Skin reactions : Rash, pruritus, and phototoxicity have occurred with the skin. Patients should avoid overexposure to sunlight or ultraviolet light while under treatment.

Musculoskeletal effects : Fluoroquinolones, including ciprofloxacin, have been connected with tendonitis and tendon rupture, most speculated with the Achilles tendon. Risk is increased in persons older than 60 years, in patients taking corticosteroids, and in individuals receiving kidney, heart or lung transplants.

Cardiovascular effects: Ciprofloxacin can prolong the QT interval, leading to an increased risk of arrhythmias. This is particularly important in patients with pre-existing heart conditions or those taking other medications that can prolong the QT interval.

Hepatic effects : Abnormal liver function tests, hepatitis, and liver failure have been reported, although these are rare.

Although serious side effects are very few, they may be so dangerous that they may need urgent medical care. These serious side effects include:

Tendon rupture: Having already pointed out this aspect, the rupture of the tendon more notably, in the Achilles tendon is a serious risk resulting from the administration of ciprofloxacin. The symptoms include sudden sharp pain in the affected tendon, swelling, and limping.

Serious hypersensitivity reactions: These could manifest as an anaphylaxis tendency, a severe allergic reaction to medicine characterized by intolerance of food taken earlier; affects breathing, swelling of the face and throat, and a drop in blood pressure. Other hypersensitivity reactions that feature are Stevens-Johnson syndrome and toxic epidermal necrolysis, which are both life-threatening conditions related to the skin.

Clostridioides difficile-associated diarrhea (CDAD): Ciprofloxacin may cause the over-proliferation of Clostridioides difficile responsible for the manifestations of severe diarrhea and colitis. CDAD may appear in the light form, but it can range upwards to the fatal stage of colitis.

Peripheral neuropathy: The reception of ciprofloxacin in some cases may cause peripheral neuropathy, manifested as numbness, tingling, or pain in the extremities. In some cases, it can be irreversible.

CNS effects: On very rare occasions, ciprofloxacin can lead to severe CNS effects, including seizures, psychosis, and heightened intracranial pressure. Patients with a history of epilepsy or any other disorders of the CNS are at a higher risk.

CHAPTER ONE

Warnings and Precautions

Tendinitis and tendon rupture: It should be advised that ciprofloxacin should be stopped straight away in case the patient experiences tendon pain, swelling, or inflammation and to avoid exercising with the affected dispersion altogether until the diagnosis of tendinitis or tendon rupture gets excluded.

Hypersensitivity reactions: Explain to patients how to recognize symptoms of hypersensitivity and measure to be taken in case of its occurrence and also recommend it to be reported straight away to a health care provider.

Photosensitivity: The patient should be cautioned against excessive exposure to sunlight or UV during treatment. Clothing and sunscreens should be advised always.

QT prolongation: The drug should be used with caution in those with pre-existing cardiac diseases, those concurrently taking drugs known to cause prolonged QT interval. Potentially altering electrolyte balance.

Peripheral neuropathy: The patient should be informed about the low risk concerning the development of peripheral neuropathy with immediate reporting of any numbness, tingling, or weakness.

Drug Interactions

Ciprofloxacin interacts with the majority of the drugs by changing their drug effects or by increasing the risk of their adverse drug effects. Some of them are as follows:

Antacids and multivitamins: The medicines which contain magnesium, aluminum, calcium, iron, or zinc chemically attach to ciprofloxacin in the gastrointestinal tract and reduce their absorption and hence their efficacy. The patient should be advised to take ciprofloxacin at least 2 hours before or 6 hours after these products.

Theophylline: Ciprofloxacin can elevate the plasma concentration of theophylline, used as a therapeutic agent in respiratory conditions like asthma and COPD, resulting in more risk of theophylline toxicity up to and including seizures and arrhythmias.

Warfarin: Ciprofloxacin can potentiate the action of warfarin in order to increase the chances of anticoagulant activity, thereby raising the tendency of bleeding. Patients taking warfarin should receive the closest possible monitoring of their INR (International Normalized Ratio) status when therapy with.

Cyclosporine: Administered concomitantly with ciprofloxacin will further increase the risk of nephrotoxicity. It is advisable to monitor renal function during treatment.

Nonsteroidal anti-inflammatory agents: Concomitant use of agents from this class with ciprofloxacin will increase the risk for CNS stimulation and possible seizures.

Corticosteroids: Administering ciprofloxacin with corticosteroid drugs increases risks of tendonitis and tendon rupture for elderly patients.

Resistance and Stewardship

Ciprofloxacin resistance in bacteria is facilitated through several means, some of which are very potent at rendering the drug relatively less efficacious. These include those :

DNA gyrase and topoisomerase IV mutations: Mutations within the genes encoding DNA gyrase and topoisomerase IV tend to decrease the binding affinity of ciprofloxacin and, therefore, resistance.

Efflux Pumps: In some cases, bacteria acquire or overexpress a class of proteins called the efflux pumps, which actively efflux ciprofloxacin from the bacterial cell, thereby reducing its intracellular concentration and hampering its activity.

Plasmid-mediated resistance: Plasmid-mediated resistance conveys resistance but can be transferred between bacteria. Plasmid-mediated resistance spreads the resistance to ciprofloxacin, and an example is the qnr gene encoding a protein that protects the DNA helicase or gyrase from being inhibited by ciprofloxacin.

Global Trends in Ciprofloxacin Resistance

Worldwide, there have been reports of ciprofloxacin resistance developed in various pathogenic strains of bacteria, and the trends have great public health concerns. Some of the prominent trends are:

Gram-negative bacteria, notably Escherichia coli and Klebsiella pneumoniae, are associated with an increasing resistance to ciprofloxacin, particularly in instances of cutaneous infections, in regions or countries with a massive antibiotic use.

Pseudomonas aeruginosa is an opportunistic pathogen and has increasingly shown resistance to ciprofloxacin, complicating the treatment of infections like pneumonia acquired in the hospital and related to.

Neisseria gonorrhoeae: The resistance to ciprofloxacin by N. gonorrhoeae has reached such a level in which the guidelines for gonorrhea treatment have been changed, so the use of other antibiotics is advised.

Mycobacterium tuberculosis: Fluoroquinolone resistance, including resistance to ciprofloxacin, is a cause for major alarm in MDR-T

The antibacterial use of ciprofloxacin and other bacterial agents should be optimized as a strategy in the fight against resistance and to help in the preservation of the effectiveness of the already available treatments. Other important key strategies are:

Healthcare providers should use ciprofloxacin with indicated, evidence-based guidelines.

Optimizing dosage: ciprofloxacin, when dosed at appropriate doses and therapy duration, minimizes adverse effects and reduces the risk of the emergence of resistance.

Culture and sensitivity testing: Culture and sensitivity testing to an antibiotic to document that the bacterial isolate is sensitive to the drug being considered always should be performed if possible and always when prescribing ciprofloxacin to be sure that it is an appropriate intervention for a given infection.

Education and awareness: Enhanced awareness of clinicians and patients about the risks of resistance and antibiotic utilization and education about proper use of antibiotics are crucial for stewardship to be successful.

Future Directions and Research

Continued efforts are underway for research into newer formulations and drug delivery methods for ciprofloxacin to make it more efficacious or reduce side effects or to better target some infections. For example:

Liposomal formulations: In this regard, it would be encapsulated within liposomes, thereby promoting directly delivery to the lungs and reducing systemic side effects.

Inhalable ciprofloxacin: Inhalable forms of ciprofloxacin are under investigation for respiratory infections, mainly in those patients who have cystic fibrosis or COPD.

Combination Therapies

Another research area directed at overcoming resistance, which focuses on improving treatment success, is the addition of ciprofloxacin to other antibiotics or adjuvant treatments. The main combinations could involve:

Ciprofloxacin and Beta-Lactam Antibiotics: Combination of

ciprofloxacin with different beta-lactam antibiotics is assumed to cause significant potentiation of antibacterial activity, especially toward.

Ciprofloxacin and efflux pump inhibitors: An efflux pump inhibitor with the administration of ciprofloxacin might enhance its efficacy against the resistant bacteria since the elimination of the antibiotic from the bacterial cell would be stopped.

Ciprofloxacin with immunomodulatory agents: The combination of ciprofloxacin and immunomodulatory agents could enhance the possibility of the host in clearance of infection and hence reduce the opportunity for the development of resistance.

Addressing Resistance

Some strategies to be employed to tackle ciprofloxacin resistance include the following:

Surveillance: Continual monitoring of the resistance patterns is advisable to track the trends and guide the treatment policy.

Novel agents: Involving new antibiotic agents, which might not be affected by ciprofloxacin resistance, is great. The approaches should include coming up with totally new classes of antibiotics and modifying old drugs.

Resistance-breaking strategies: For example, phage therapy—targeting resistant bacteria with the help of bacteriophages—and the CRISPR-Cas system are used for the destruction of resistance genes. These are under research for use as alternate treatment strategies to combat antibiotic resistance.

Conclusion

Ciprofloxacin is still, however, a very useful antibiotic with a wide spectrum of activity and a broad range of clinical applications. This antibiotic has proved highly effective against a broad range of bacterial pathogens and has really become the bedrock of modern antibiotic therapy. On the other hand, the occurrence of resistance and several serious side effects further reiterate that ciprofloxacin should be used judiciously within the concept of antimicrobial stewardship programs.

As research progresses, new formulations, delivery methods, and combination therapies may improve the utility of ciprofloxacin while risk-mitigating. Combating the challenge of antibacterial resistance will, hence, need a combined commitment among care providers, researchers, and public health policymakers to ensure that ciprofloxacin and other antibiotics tools remain effective in fighting bacterial infections.

THE END

www.ingramcontent.com/pod-product-compliance
Lightning Source LLC
Chambersburg PA
CBHW030055230526
45471CB00003B/1102